ENDORSEMENTS

This book is an extraordinary resource for anyone faced with navigating the decisions involved with being a caregiver. The simplicity of this text is perfect for loved ones who are already overwhelmed by the reality of supporting a sick patient. It is rich with practical advice while also conveying compassion for the caregiver. From the perspective of a physician working with chronically ill patients and their families for over fifteen years now, I highly recommend this book for family members and friends caring for their loved ones.

—Dr. Katie Dahlgren

Caregiving is a challenging task, and understanding the world of hospitals and clinics may be particularly challenging. Ms. Gold has written a concise, practical guide to help caregivers navigate hospital stays and doctor visits. This guide allows caregivers to prepare for questions likely to be asked and understand the process of admission and medical visits. Understanding these processes allows caregivers to feel less stressed when they know what to expect.

—Dr. Kristine Rinn

The process of hospital care can be complex and sensitive when a loved one is in the hospital with multifaceted issues or facing end-of-life questions. It is important to have tools and resources available. Jody Gold does a wonderful job of balancing the difficulties of these issues with compassion. Her personal experience shines through like a guide. There are so many practical, hands-on tools for a caregiver or loved one to put into immediate use. I encourage everyone to have this guide handy so you can have what you need to focus on the care needed.

—Sadie Hess, founder and CEO, Compass Supported and Independent Living Services

Jody has a heart of gold as an advocate for giving excellence in care and ultimately value for individuals being supported. This caregiver's guide holds to the heart of the needs of those being served, and it maintains their dignity while enabling and creating a space for those professionals to use their skills and also learn the individual in front of them. I am pleased to endorse this material, as it comes from the heart of someone who cares and has had loved ones who have needed this very support. Thank you for your courage to change the world around us.

—Josh Flom, regional manager, Compass Far North

What a great guidebook this is. A much-needed and easy-to-use roadmap that facilitates communication between caregivers, patients, and hospital staff, enabling the best possible care for the patient or loved one. This guide provides the ability to have all the patient information pre-collected in one place, which can make intake much easier. It also provides sections for capturing ongoing information, as well as suggestions for actions by the caregiver during and after the patient's hospital visit. By being organized, the caregiver can focus more time on ensuring the patient or loved one is comfortable and safe.

—Don and Bobbi Hascall, parents and grandparents, caring for those in the community

Many people enter the acute inpatient setting with little or no experience navigating through acute inpatient care and insurance barriers and coordinating the least restrictive post-acute settings. The ability to learn and adapt to these new systems is often compromised by the emotional toll of the illness or injury a loved one is experiencing, and further confounded by the acronym-rich dialect health-care workers speak. A guide like this provides an overview, helps identify who in a hospital can help with specific concerns, offers reference points for questions, clarifies hospital roles for caregivers, and offers helpful skills and tricks to better manage expectations and effectively advocate for a loved one.

—Theodore Lynch, LCSW, care coordination, manager of social work

The
CAREGIVER'S
QUICK GUIDE
to MEDICAL CARE

The CAREGIVER'S QUICK GUIDE *to* MEDICAL CARE

HOW TO NAVIGATE HOSPITAL CARE,
COMMUNICATION, AND SERVICES

JODY L. GOLD

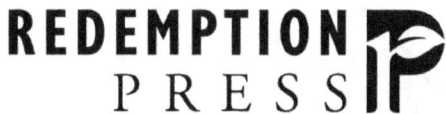
REDEMPTION PRESS

ISBN 13: 978-1-951350-60-4
Library of Congress Catalog Card Number: 2023915858

Dedication

This book is dedicated to the beautiful souls of the world who are caregivers, without whom patients would have a very different quality of life. To my late mother, Kathleen Wells, and my late brother, Matt Davison, both of whom experienced the kindness and compassion from caregivers during a time when the world was locked down and family was prohibited in the hospital. I am grateful beyond words. I have the greatest amount of respect for caregivers and the medical community at large. Your kindness is so needed in this world today.
With immense gratitude.

ACKNOWLEDGMENTS

I am endlessly grateful to those who have so graciously allowed me to learn and grow through my experience while being part of a larger purpose.

I want to profoundly thank my editor, Victoria M., for her professional skills and such attention to detail. I would be lost without her. To my ghostwriter, who is extremely talented and a gifted artist. Her elegance with words brings art to life. Thanks to Anne G. To my coach, Zina, who was vital during the challenging and victorious moments. She has taught me to celebrate every win, even the smallest ones. I truly couldn't have reached the finish line without her next to me.

I am thankful for the staff at Compass Cares. They provide services for adults with disabilities in Northern California. They were instrumental in providing a team of support day and night. The communication and level of care were first rate.

Mercy Medical Center in conjunction with Dignity Health provided the knowledge and dedication to their patients that goes above and beyond the standard of care. I could not have stood in calm during a major storm without them.

While the list is vast, I would be remiss not to mention Katie at Compass for her intentional kindness and love that went far beyond her position. Ted, a social worker at Mercy Hospital, who saw through to the human spirit keeping open the process to preserve dignity. I felt that, and it mattered so much. Shannon in palliative care at Mercy Hospital treated me like a family member who had serious decisions to make. Your level of kindness and guidance I shall not forget. Tanya, a care coordinator at Mercy Hospital, showed so much grace and understanding of the position I was in. She was the guiding light of hope who showed me that I wasn't alone. A special thank-you to notary public Pamela, who not only made house calls but handled sensitive subject matter and explained it with precise care. Her patience and understanding found me in tears of joy. Allen and Dahl Funeral Chapel, who virtually held my hands and heart together, twice. An odd time for finding closure remotely. You were such a blessing.

Last, I am profoundly grateful for all those who kept our family in prayer.

To those of you who will intentionally take this guide, this was a labor of love, and my hope is that it will serve you well in the comfort and care of those you protect. It matters so much.

CONTENTS

FOREWORD

This guide that you hold in your hands is the result of the real-life experiences Jody encountered while caring for her mother and then taking over the mantle to care for her disabled brother after her mom's passing. A labor of love, born out of the grief of losing two family members while navigating the maze of medical care. You will find, just as Jody did, that there are many compassionate and caring people in the health-care system, and they are overwhelmed. Being even just a little bit prepared will not only help you, but it will also help the health-care staff provide the best care possible.

Whether you are a professional or personal caregiver, this guide will provide practical, sound advice that you can use while navigating the medical care system. A path to follow in the midst of situations that can be emotionally overwhelming. Having an idea of what to do next, whom to talk to, or what questions to ask, will allow you to focus more time on your patient or loved one and ensure they are receiving the best care possible.

Knowing the author as I do, I can tell you that Jody's sincerest wish is that you can make use of this guide to enable you to focus on the well-being of your patient or loved one and find comfort in knowing that someone has done this before and understands what you are going through.

Love always,

Glenn Gold
Husband, father, caregiver

INTRODUCTION

When a patient or loved one with or without disabilities is in the hospital, there are many choices that need to be made. From the moment they are admitted until they are discharged, caregivers can influence the type of care the patient will receive.

Hospital care is subjective depending on the situation and the patient. The caregiver can explain what the patient would want should they not be able to verbally express it. The caregiver is an intermediary for the patient, expressing to the hospital staff what the patient needs.

During the process of caregiving, many things will influence your decisions. As a caregiver, you know the specific needs of the person. You will also be acutely aware of what they like and don't like as far as their daily care is concerned.

Often in serious situations, a care coordinator is assigned to the family. Each patient may be assigned a care coordinator or a case manager RN. In addition to the services they provide, they are responsible for coordination and review with insurance companies for the purpose of securing acute care on a case-by-case basis. Note: this may vary by state and location. Be sure to check with the facilities in your area.

The care coordinator is familiar with many scenarios that happen during a hospital stay and the services that are accessible to each patient. The advice they give should be taken seriously and with great thought as to the next steps in the patient's care.

The care coordinator is also directly involved in the after-hospital stay. With your input, they can influence and work directly with various agencies that will be most beneficial to the patient after being discharged from the hospital. The care coordinator has relationships with many of the care facilities and rehabilitation centers, as well as with palliative care providers and end-of-life care. This person will be your go-between from the nursing staff and doctors to social services.

You should ask for the name of the care coordinator assigned to the patient; it is imperative that you find out who this person is as soon as possible.

The next step, depending on the patient's situation, would be to contact social services. Think of the caregiver, care coordinator, and hospital staff as a team put in place for the comfort and care of the patient.

In instances where a patient is also in the care of another entity, such as a care facility, it is important to establish contact with the person in charge of their care at that facility. If you are facilitating care between the hospital and a care facility, you will need to take steps to ensure that all communication between the hospital and care facility is carefully documented. Have a notebook to keep track of who you spoke to and when.

There are pages at the end of this guide with spaces for questions and answers, which will be very important in the days to come. You'll need to contact many of these people multiple times. Having all the information documented will give you the opportunity to review all the details. This will allow for reflection and help to clarify what steps to take next.

I have found that the kinder you are to all the parties involved, the better the results. These are kind and caring people, but there will be some who are more difficult to deal with than others. It is important to remember that your patient or loved one is not the only person in their care. Each time you call, you should give your name, relationship to the patient, name of the patient, and room number if you have it. This will get you the information you need about your patient or loved one in a timely manner. The patient's information is kept on a whiteboard at the nurse's station, so they can quickly identify the nurse in charge when you provide the room number and the patient's name. This method of displayed information may vary by hospital and location.

While it's important to ask a lot of questions, it's equally important to write down the answers so that you do not ask the same question again. I cannot stress enough that there are many patients being taken care of, and it is much easier for the attending nurses if they don't have to repeat themselves.

By keeping notes, you can also update the current nurse about a prior conversation with another staff member if necessary.

If your patient or loved one is having an extended stay, it is in your best interest to give the nurses your name and phone number should they need to contact you. If you live out of state, be sure to also include the area code. They do not have the time to look in a file or find a phone message. However, they are usually very happy to tell you how your patient or loved one is doing.

There are no questions that are unacceptable to ask. If a relationship with the nurses has been established, I've found them excited and more than willing to share positive progress with you.

Before the hospital is ready to discharge the patient, the discussion with the care coordinator will include what kind of services the patient may need for their ongoing recovery. There is a wide range of services for rehabilitation and after-hospital care. Keep in mind, the continuation of care must be prescribed *before* the patient is discharged from the hospital in most cases. Here are a few therapies that may apply after discharge: neurological therapy, physical therapy, occupational therapy, geriatric physical therapy, rehabilitative physical therapy, hand physical therapy, and speech therapy. Home health social work is also common.

The crucial thing here is that the services need to be ordered by the discharging doctor to avoid the challenges of getting a prescription after discharge. An active conversation with the doctor regarding follow-up care will be needed. Doctors are busy, so you may need to ask the nurse to inform the doctor of your request for a quick conversation when they visit the patient's room. When the doctor, nurses, and facilitators feel that you are an active part of the care solutions for the patient, they are more willing to take the time to discuss in detail what the patient may need next. The more you know and are involved in the process, the better prepared you are for the next steps in care.

What is the process to obtain the patient's medical records should you need them? First, to have that access, you must have a copy of the power of attorney (POA) for health care, which will need to be either notarized or signed by two witnesses (check your state and local laws for verification). This document states which individuals have been given power by the patient to authorize any copying of their records. Second, most medical facilities require a form called a Release of Information (ROI), which they provide for you to fill out to indicate your status. The POA should be attached to this ROI form.

This is also true for the primary care doctor or facility to provide any records. This process is best done in person. However, each hospital and medical facility has a records department you can call to find out the procedure that is in place. After a hospital visit, the primary care doctor receives the information related to the visit electronically.

CURRENT PATIENT INFORMATION AND ALLERGIC REACTION ALERTS

T he current patient information form should be filled out ahead of the hospital visit. This important sheet will be with the patient so details can be relayed without delay to the staff. The ER doctor has the ability to contact the primary care doctor by phone during normal business hours if they have specific questions. Be sure to include the primary care doctor's direct phone number.

An additional copy of this form is included in the appendix for your convenience.

CURRENT PATIENT INFORMATION
AND ALLERGIC REACTIONS

Patient's name: _____

Patient prefers to be called: _____

Patient's primary care doctor: _____

Phone number: _____

Name of family member to contact: _____

Phone:_____ Date contacted: _____

Baseline (check all that apply and describe assistance needed):

( ) CPAP _____

( ) Wheelchair _____

( ) Speech delayed _____

( ) Bathroom assistance _____

( ) Diabetic _____

( ) Add anything not listed:

A. _____ B. _____

Current medications and schedule of time taken below (example: Citalopram 2x daily a.m. and p.m. with food):

1._____ 2. _____

3._____ 4. _____

5._____ 6. _____

Supplements: _____

Special dietary needs (e.g., gluten /dairy intolerance): _____

Patient allergies (include life-threatening allergies):

1._____

2. _____

INITIAL HOSPITAL INTAKE INFORMATION

These items are for hospital intake. I've included below a list of items that will be most important for you to keep track of each time you speak to the hospital. Be sure to write down the date and the name of the nurse you spoke with each time as well.

Important: POA forms can be found online, and they are specific by state. You will need one for the state the patient resides in and it must be notarized or signed by two witnesses to be valid. Refer to your state's probate code for applicability of witness signatures. Ideally, this would be done before the patient is admitted. If it is being completed in a skilled nursing facility (SNF), the ombudsman (see definition in terms) must be present at the time of signing.

In contemplation of the patient's desires for end-of-life treatment, consider using a POLST (Physician Orders for Life-Sustaining Treatment) form. Check with your primary care physician for more information.

An initial hospital intake form is shown here; an additional copy of this form is included in the appendix for your convenience.

INITIAL HOSPITAL INTAKE INFORMATION

Name of hospital: _____

Date admitted: _____ Time: _____

Patient's name and room #: _____

Your name: _____

Your relationship to the patient: _____

Your phone #: _____

Power of attorney for health care: YES _____ NO _____

Does patient have a POLST (Physician Orders for Life-Sustaining Treatment)?

YES _____ NO _____ (Important: See definition in terms.)

Does the patient have a DNR (Do Not Resuscitate) order? YES _____ NO _____

(Important: See definition in terms.)

Name of doctor: _____

Name of nurse: _____

Hospital sitter name (if applicable): _____

Care facility (if there is one): _____

Date of admission to care facility: _____

Care coordinator's name at hospital and date: _____

Social services contact name: _____

Is there online access to medical records? YES ___ NO ___

If yes, sign-in and password: _____

Medical card / insurance information: _____

_____

Patient's current pharmacy: _____

Transport/ambulance company (if not transported by you): _____

DAILY CALL AND CHECK-IN

When the caregiver accompanies the patient for multiple days, at the hospital or checking in with the hospital by phone, it is imperative to have a place to keep all the information about the patient. This can also include communications with after-care facilities. This daily call and check-in sheet will keep the patient's information in one convenient place. When the time comes to relay the information to the care facility, or a family member, or caregiver, it will all be in one place.

See the next page for the daily call and check-in sheet. Multiple copies of this sheet are available for your convenience in the appendix.

DAILY CALL AND CHECK-IN SHEET

Date of call: _____

Patient's name and room number: _____

Your relationship to the patient: _____

Name of doctor: _____

Name of nurse: _____

Hospital care coordinator: _____

Social services contact: _____

Questions I have for the doctor or nurse:

Question: _____

Answer: _____

Question: _____

Answer: _____

Question: _____

Answer: _____

Notes:

TIME-SAVING TIPS

When calling the hospital

Make sure to identify yourself. For example: "My name is Barbara Stone, from the Compass Facility. I am calling to speak to the nurse for room 201. The patient is Mark Ross." Please note, the patient can be moved at any time depending on how many patient beds are needed. You will not know ahead of time if the room number changes, so it is important to write it down for your next call. Always leave your name, relationship to the patient, and phone number so you can be reached for any reason.

Current medication list from home

Be sure to have the list of medications ready when you call in case you need to reference them to the doctor. Typically, medications do not travel to the hospital with the patient. In some cases, the current pharmacy can provide assistance if they are made aware of the request. However, it is critical that the doctor knows what medications the patient is taking and the dosage. The hospital can get necessary medications quickly for the patient if they have access to this information.

The primary care physician

Have the current name and phone number of the doctor primarily caring for the patient on a regular basis. This will save the hospital physician the time of looking it up if they need to call for any reason.

Checking patient status

Write down your questions ahead of time the best you can. By letting the doctor know you have questions right away, they can be addressed before the doctor has to attend to the next patient. Doctors and nurses care for multiple patients and have limited time. Be sure to write down their answers too.

Medication for home care

It is easier for the caregiver to ask if the new medications can be filled at the hospital *before* the patient is discharged. This saves the extra step and frustration of having to drop off the prescription at the pharmacy with the patient and waiting to pick it up before continuing home. Being discharged from the hospital can sometimes be a lengthy process, so this should give the pharmacy enough time to fill the prescriptions to be taken home. In addition, with prescriptions in hand, calling the pharmacy before leaving the hospital can also help if the insurance requires prior authorization. Be sure to ask ahead of time.

HOSPITAL NAVIGATION

The goal is to provide as much important information as possible about the patient to the hospital. This will enable the hospital to provide quality care to the patient or your loved one based on their specific needs. Never assume the hospital will know about every situation. Each person has their individual needs and preferences.

Understanding how the hospital team works will save everyone time when exchanging information about the patient. The nurses change shifts early in the morning, midafternoon, and late in the evening. However, shift changes can vary based on state and location. When getting an update on the patient, the nurses will often refer to information left in the patient's chart by staff on a previous shift. For longer stays, it really helps to build a rapport with the staff. It helps them to know that you support them and are concerned about the comfort and care of the patient.

The more you know about the inner workings of how the hospital and staff work together, the more comfortable you will be with all the aspects involved in caregiving and advocating for the patient or your loved one. Everyone is working together to make sure the patient is understood and their needs are communicated, even if they cannot communicate clearly or at all. You are their voice, and you have the information about what they prefer. It is imperative that you communicate this to the staff on behalf of the patient. This may have to be done multiple times.

SPECIAL CIRCUMSTANCES

An important communication tool for the hospital staff is posting instructions above the patient's bed. Because my disabled brother could not clearly communicate his needs, I asked the nurse to post the following above his bed:

Matt is mentally delayed at baseline.

His behavior is not malicious.

He is scared and confused.

Please speak slowly and clearly.

Thank you!

This term *baseline* is vital for a disabled, elderly, or infirm patient. It gives the hospital staff the ability to measure a patient's progress with the starting point being their status when they enter the hospital.

Things that the patient needs in their daily care routine, or things that are part of the patient's specific needs should be relayed to the hospital staff by the caregiver upon admission to the hospital. Some examples of this include: Does the patient use equipment at home, such as a wheelchair or a CPAP machine? Does the patient need bathroom assistance? Is the patient's speech delayed?

Before they enter the hospital, it is vitally important for you to communicate these items to the staff so that, during the times you are not with the patient, the staff has a full understanding of the capabilities and/or disabilities of the patient. This knowledge will allow them to care for the patient or your loved one accordingly.

If the caregiver cannot be with the patient overnight, you can ask for a sitter to be in the room. The sitter would also need to be informed of the patient's baseline needs. A sitter is often used for patients who are confused, a fall risk, impulsive, or likely to injure themselves or staff due to confusion. Additionally, they may be uncomfortable or scared. This is a good option instead of the patient being left alone. If the patient has full-time care at home, this option can be very comforting during their stay.

CELEBRATION OF LIFE, BURIAL, AND ARRANGEMENTS

This section, difficult as it may be, is information most of us do not inherently know. The person who provided many answers to me was the care coordinator at the hospital. Care coordinators have a wealth of knowledge. They, as well as chaplains and social workers, have pertinent local, state, federal, and veterans information. They will help guide you in the right direction.

There are many ways to celebrate a person's life. This is personal and often within the confines of a family and in accordance with the wishes of the patient if specified prior to the patient's passing. If a power of attorney for health care is in place or the patient has a will, this information may be covered. If you are a family member, you would most likely have an idea of what the person would want.

Having this in mind, a caregiver may not have all the up-to-date information. When engaging in conversation, the care coordinator will ask a series of questions that will help determine the direction they will provide. One of the things I did not know for burial is that a person with a disability diagnosed by a doctor before the age of eighteen can be placed with a veteran family member if certain qualifications are met.

In my case, my mother was placed with her husband, who was a veteran. These were her wishes. However, there was nothing in place for my disabled brother when he passed. During an emotional conversation with the care coordinator, she advised me that since my brother was disabled and I had supporting information to that effect, my brother could be placed with my mom at the veteran's cemetery. The family was laid to rest together. This made the other aspects of the process a bit easier.

The funeral home had a vast amount of specific information pertaining to the next steps. Because I was out of state, this was all done by phone.

If a patient is disabled, they may be receiving state or federal assistance. This can complicate matters because outside companies often take care of the financial piece away from the actual care facility, and the care services may be provided at home or in a facility.

As a family member, you may not have access to this critical information. The power of attorney for health care will indicate who has that access. It is imperative to get power of attorney should you be responsible for decisions pertaining to the patient's health care.

The funeral home is a neutral go-between and should be utilized. Most companies will work together so you can find a resolution to the services needed for the burial, celebration of life, or final arrangements. The coordination between these entities can be a time-consuming process.

As a side note, be aware that the chaplain can be contacted at any time for emotional and spiritual support. They can provide support to not just the patient but to friends and family as well. I found this to be comforting to both the patient and the family. These are some of the most compassionate and caring people you will ever meet.

GRIEF SUPPORT

A grief counselor may help in finding your way after the loss of a loved one. Contact human resources to see if you have benefits through your employer. An online program for grief support was sent to me by the funeral home after my brother passed. This was called grief.everythingafter.com. This service consisted of prerecorded videos of therapists addressing every aspect of pain, grief, anger, compassion, and much more. Since it was online, it was accessible from anywhere.

The beautiful thing about online grief support is that you can move through the process with your feelings and emotions in private. You can watch what pertains to you specifically whenever you need. I found this to be extremely helpful, and I still have access to it today.

I highly recommend seeking out support either online or by contacting your local pastor, chaplain, or a social worker. If you prefer an in-person group setting, be sure to share that with the professional you contact. It may be helpful to talk with others going through a similar situation. Grief shows up in different forms for each of us.

My heart is full of compassion for anyone who is experiencing the pain of losing a loved one. Please don't think you have to do it alone. There is an extensive amount of support and grief services available.

CONCLUSION

These are some things I learned going through the grieving process of two loved ones who passed close together. The emotions experienced during grief cannot be controlled. Things will come up that you never imagined. Losing my mother brought up childhood and family memories of all sorts. Losing my brother, who was two years younger than I, brought up many memories of the experiences we had. There is much to be thankful for. The flip side is that pain and a sense of loss are inevitable.

How you choose to get through your grief is uniquely your process. There is no right or wrong way to grieve. Be patient with yourself. A timetable for grief does not exist. There are times I feel like I have moved forward in so many ways. At other times, memories will rush over me, catching me off guard.

Palm tree

I've been known to keep palm trees alive in my house throughout the years of harsh, cold Pacific Northwest weather. The one in my office sits just at my eyeline and reflects green glowing energy back to me when I need inspiration. I look to it and appreciate the sheer beauty of life that accompanies me in my most sacred space day in and day out.

Over the last three or so years, the palm tree had started to wilt and shrug off some of the energy it usually carries. Maybe I'd neglected a watering or two or kept the shades down for too many days in a row. It now reflected how I felt inside: neglected, dissatisfied, abandoned. I noticed myself starting to wilt and lean up against structures when I couldn't hold myself up. I realized we both were missing vital parts of survival.

As I nurtured my palm back to healthy life, I took cautious care to give my own soul what it needed to come back to life. I had to respond with kindness and intention when it came to putting the light back in my eyes.

Now I see the lesson in the palm that I so deeply cherish. I can give light, I can be light, I can grow, and I can be alive to my fullest extent *only* when my cup is full. The best way I can love the people and things around me is when I love myself first. Now every time I water my palm tree, it's a reminder, nay, a reflection of watering myself.

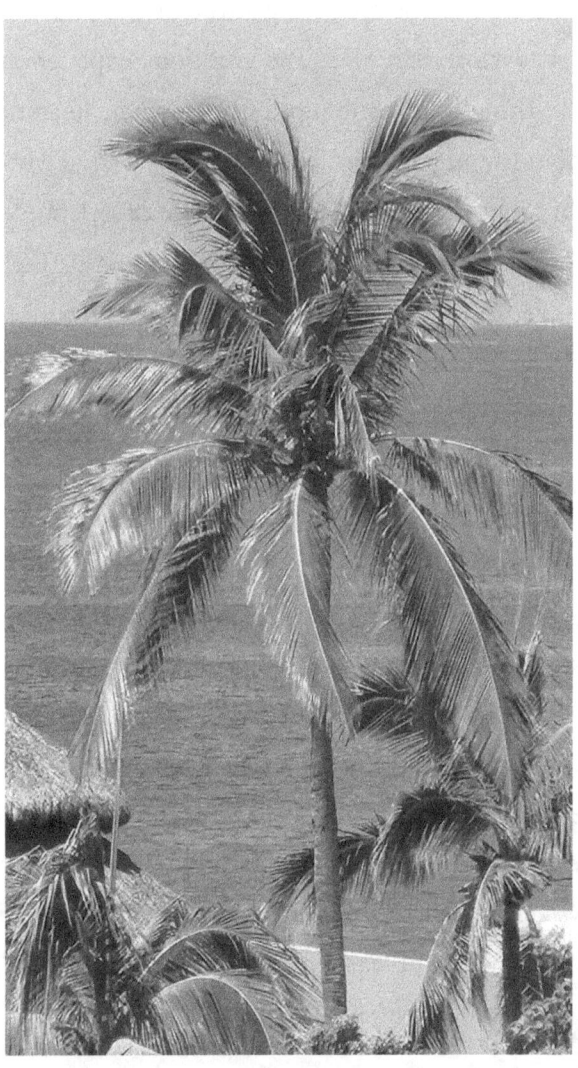

APPENDIX

DEFINITION OF TERMS

Celebration of life. A memorial service that is performed without the remains of the deceased person present in a coffin or urn. (See also funeral.)

Comfort care. *Palliative care*, *supportive care*, and *hospice care* are terms used for end-of-life care. Palliative care is alleviation of suffering, which can also be provided outside of end-of-life/comfort care.

CPAP machine. Continuous positive airway pressure. A form of ventilation in which a constant level of pressure greater than atmospheric pressure is continuously applied to the upper respiratory tract of a person.

DNR. Do not resuscitate. An order previously written and signed by the patient indicating that they do not want CPR performed in the event their heart should stop beating. Requirements for this document vary by state. It is important that all medical personnel are aware that the patient has a DNR order in place.

Disabled person. A person with a physical or developmental difference or someone with a behavioral or emotional difference. These may include but are not limited to individuals with autism, cerebral palsy, Down syndrome, dyslexia, dyscalculia, dyspraxia, dysgraphia, blindness, deafness, ADHD, and cystic fibrosis.

Funeral. A funeral is a spiritual ceremony to honor, memorialize, and celebrate an individual with a casketed body present during the service.

Geriatric therapy. Focuses on the unique movement needs of older adults.

Grief services. See Support.

Hand therapy. Focuses on the art and science of rehabilitation of the upper limb, which includes the hand, wrist, elbow, and shoulder girdle.

Hospital chaplain. Offers spiritual guidance and pastoral care to patients and their families. As representatives of various religious traditions, chaplains in hospitals and medical centers use the insights and principles of psychology, religion, spirituality, and theology.

Hospital sitter. Provides one-on-one supervision for safety issues such as falls, impulsiveness, suicidality, confusion, etc. Compassionate care in hospital before and after treatment.

Long-term care. Facilities include nursing homes, rehabilitation facilities, inpatient behavioral health, and long-term chronic hospitals.

Medical records. Documents that explain all details about the patient's history, clinical findings, diagnostic test results, pre- and postoperative care, progress, and medication.

Neurological therapy. Focuses on the treatment of movement problems related to disease or injury of the nervous system.

Occupational therapy. Helps injured, ill, or disabled patients by practicing everyday activities such as brushing teeth, getting dressed, and eating.

Ombudsman. A person who investigates, reports on, and helps settle complaints. An individual usually affiliated with an organization or business who serves as an advocate, for patients in this case. A trained advocate for residents of nursing and rest homes.

Definition of Terms

Orthopedic therapy. Focuses on restoring function to the musculoskeletal system, including joints, tendons, ligaments, and bones.

Pediatric therapy. Focuses on determining where delays or limitations are coming from, especially in the areas of fine motor skills, cognitive skills, social development, and establishing self-care routines.

Physical therapies. Ongoing methods used to preserve, enhance, or restore physical functions damaged or threatened by illness or accident. (See also orthopedic therapy, geriatric therapy, neurological therapy, occupational therapy, hand therapy, pediatric therapy.)

POA. Power of attorney for health care. A document required to speak on behalf of a patient as far as ongoing care, comfort, and continued services. Ideally, this would be done ahead of time to discuss what choices the patient would want for care if they cannot advocate for themselves.

Note: As an example, California Probate Code 4701 Section (5.3) Statement of Witnesses provides guidance as to the requirements for witness signatures vs. notarization.

This may vary from state to state.

Additional Note: There are numerous types of POAs that cover different things. If the focus is health care, a power of attorney for health care or an advanced directive makes sense. Many people are interested in paying for a loved one's bills or managing their finances while they are in the hospital. They would need to complete a general POA or have a trust in place and follow the steps to transition the executor from the patient to the first alternate. Check the provisions for the state in which the patient resides.

Physician Orders for Life-Sustaining Treatment (POLST). This form is a written medical order from a physician, nurse practitioner, or physician assistant to help give people with serious illnesses more control over their own care by specifying the types of medical treatment they want to receive during serious illness. This is a tool for end of life. Note: These forms are state specific and can be accessed by looking under the state the patient resides in.

Rehabilitation facility. Often the next step in care after the patient has been stabilized and released from the hospital. These facilities may include rehabilitation for neurological, musculoskeletal, orthopedic, and other medical conditions after a hospital stay.

Rehabilitation care. There are two types of acute rehabilitation:
1. Three+ hours per day of at least two types of therapy, usually a ten- to fourteen-day stay.
2. Placement at a skilled nursing facility (less than three hours of therapy per day but with routine stays of two to three weeks that can extend to a few months or convert into custodial/long-term care).

Release of Information (ROI). Authorization for release of information. The form prescribed by the agency for the purpose of authorizing the release of a confidential record, signed and dated by the person empowered to release the information.

Skilled nursing facility (SNF). A nursing facility with the staff and equipment to give skilled nursing care and/or skilled rehabilitation services and other related health services.

Speech therapy. Treatment that improves your ability to talk and use other language skills.

Social services. Often a social worker in a hospital setting will speak with you about the mental health of the patient and what services or treatment they need now and in the future. In addition to mental health, the social worker may address nonmedical needs to prevent rehospitalization, such as food, shelter, income, substance use, community programs and supports, regional services, etc.

Definition of Terms

Support: grief services. There are many different services available. The usual route is to find
a therapist who specializes in grief therapy. There are support groups available as well.
Start by accessing the five stages of grief.

CURRENT PATIENT INFORMATION
AND ALLERGIC REACTIONS

Patient's name: _____

Patient prefers to be called: _____

Patient's primary care doctor: _____

Phone number: _____

Name of family member to contact: _____

Phone:_____ Date contacted: _____

Baseline: Check all that apply and describe assistance needed.

( ) CPAP_____

( ) Wheelchair_____

( ) Speech delayed_____

( ) Bathroom assistance _____

( ) Diabetic _____

( ) Add anything not listed:

A._____ B._____

Current medications and schedule of time taken (example: Citalopram 2x daily a.m. and p.m. with food):

1._____ 2. _____

3._____ 4. _____

5._____ 6. _____

Supplements: _____

Special dietary needs (e.g., gluten /dairy intolerance): _____

Patient allergies (including life-threatening allergies):

1._____

2. _____

INITIAL HOSPITAL INTAKE INFORMATION

Name of hospital: _____

Date admitted: _____Time: _____

Patient's name and room #: _____

Your name: _____

Your relationship to the patient: _____

Your phone #: _____

Power of attorney for health care: YES _____ NO _____

Does patient have a POLST (Physician Orders for Life-Sustaining Treatment)?
YES _____ NO _____ (Important: See definition in terms.)

Does the patient have a DNR (Do Not Resuscitate) order? YES _____ NO _____
(Important: See definition in terms.)

Name of doctor: _____

Name of nurse: _____

Hospital sitter name (if applicable): _____

Care facility (if there is one): _____

Date of admission to care facility: _____

Care coordinator's name at hospital and date: _____

Social services contact name: _____

Is there online access to medical records? YES _____ NO _____

If yes, sign-in and password: _____

Medical card/insurance information: _____

_____

Patient's current pharmacy: _____

Transport/ambulance company (if not transported by you): _____

DAILY CALL AND CHECK-IN SHEET

Date of call: _____

Patient's name and room number: _____

Your relationship to the patient: _____

Name of doctor: _____

Name of nurse: _____

Hospital care coordinator: _____

Social services contact: _____

Questions I have for the doctor or nurse:

Question: _____

Answer: _____

Question: _____

Answer: _____

Question: _____

Answer: _____

Notes on back:

DAILY CALL AND CHECK-IN SHEET

Date of call: _____

Patient's name and room number: _____

Your relationship to the patient: _____

Name of doctor: _____

Name of nurse: _____

Hospital care coordinator: _____

Social services contact: _____

Questions I have for the doctor or nurse:

Question: _____

Answer: _____

Question: _____

Answer: _____

Question: _____

Answer: _____

Notes on back:

DAILY CALL AND CHECK-IN SHEET

Date of call: _____

Patient's name and room number: _____

Your relationship to the patient: _____

Name of doctor: _____

Name of nurse: _____

Hospital care coordinator: _____

Social services contact: _____

Questions I have for the doctor or nurse:

Question: _____

Answer: _____

Question:_____

Answer: _____

Question: _____

Answer: _____

Notes on back:

DAILY CALL AND CHECK-IN SHEET

Date of call: _____

Patient's name and room number: _____

Your relationship to the patient: _____

Name of doctor: _____

Name of nurse: _____

Hospital care coordinator: _____

Social services contact: _____

Questions I have for the doctor or nurse:

Question: _____

Answer: _____

Question: _____

Answer: _____

Question: _____

Answer: _____

Notes on back:

DAILY CALL AND CHECK-IN SHEET

Date of call: _____

Patient's name and room number: _____

Your relationship to the patient: _____

Name of doctor: _____

Name of nurse: _____

Hospital care coordinator: _____

Social services contact: _____

Questions I have for the doctor or nurse:

Question: _____

Answer: _____

Question:_____

Answer: _____

Question: _____

Answer: _____

Notes on back:

ORDER INFORMATION

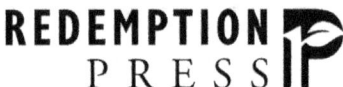

To order additional copies of this book, please visit
www.redemption-press.com.
Also available at Christian bookstores, Amazon, and Barnes and Noble.

www.ingramcontent.com/pod-product-compliance
Lightning Source LLC
Chambersburg PA
CBHW081617220526
45468CB00010B/2912